Acupuncture.

A Pain Free Approach

Gail Daugherty,

LAc, MAcOM, Board Certified Acupuncturist
(NCAAOM™), MBA, PhD (Holistic Nutrition)

Acupuncture:

A Pain Free Approach

Gail Daugherty,

LAc, MAcOM, Board Certified Acupuncturist
(NCAAOM™), MBA, PhD (Holistic Nutrition)

Table of Contents

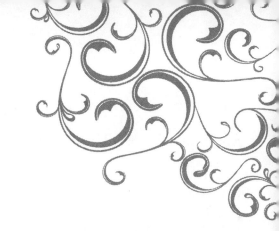

Introduction

Why Did I Stay In Pain?

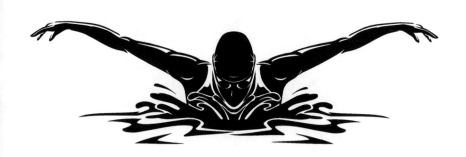

Acupuncture: A Pain Free Approach

Some days it took a five-minute conversation to prepare myself for the pain of washing and brushing my hair. Most nights were filled with tossing and turning as I tried to find a comfortable sleeping position. Having long hair and desiring sleep lead to constant frustration and tears.

I began pushing my body physically when I was six years old. I discovered that I loved and had a talent for swimming very fast. Swimming helped pay for college, taught me resilience, and made me strong. Over the years it also created a shoulder pain I could not ignore or push through. Missing months of training to help my shoulder rest and recover ruined any hope of competing in the Olympic Trials.

The pain intensified over the years, and I was losing more and more range of motion, so much that I could barely lift my arm to brush my hair. Ignoring my shoulder injury for over a decade led to excruciating pain with no relief, no sleep, and no more swimming.

The pain became constant. My shoulder would throb, ache, stab, and my hand would stay numb. It was affecting my ability to sleep soundly, to get dressed, and I was becoming a very frustrated. I was an athlete, and I believed that athletes do not give in to pain; we just keep fighting through and ignore it.

My fascination with acupuncture predates my trying it by many years. I was intrigued by the success stories I heard and in disbelief it could truly help me. My pain was bad. How could a little needle help? A fellow athlete suggested I try it, and my first thought was: No way, that's going to hurt. I did relent and try one session. It did not help. I was like most skeptics, writing off acupuncture because it didn't cure years of pain in one session.

After working for a short time as a nutritionist for a reality television show, I began teaching Biochemical Nutrition at an acupuncture school. To avoid surgery, and with the urging of my students, I eventually tried acupuncture. I was yet to be convinced it would help.

The first session wasn't at all what I expected. It was different than the first time I had tried it. In truth, I found it calming and comforting. Decades of damage was not relieved immediately, but I saw improvements within a few sessions. After months of treatments, my shoulder pain went away completely, and I regained full range of motion. That was the beginning of my love affair with traditional Chinese medicine. Thousands of years old, it is a profound healing art that truly relieves pain. It was then I decided to learn this remarkable and mysterious medicine.

Since then, I have become a licensed and board-certified acupuncturist and received my Masters in Acupuncture and Oriental Medicine. I have worked with thousands of patients and helped with hundreds of different conditions.

We tend to scoff or fear something we don't understand, like acupuncture. We are told the body is connected, but it is not demonstrated when we go to the doctor. If your knee hurts, doctors look at your knee. If your shoulder hurts, they look at your shoulder. As you will see, acupuncture follows a different approach to health. It is old, comprehensive, and effective. There have been endless studies confirming the efficacy of acupuncture. I hope to encourage even the greatest skeptic to give it a try and experience a life with less pain.

Most importantly, acupuncture can work for you as it has for thousands of years for millions of people. When writing, I was determined to give you a brief background in acupuncture, explain how acupuncture works, and let you hear from my patients who can attest to the power of acupuncture. In the end, I hope it is both informative and inspiring.

Acupuncture is a safe and effective form of holistic medicine that can be used alone or in conjunction with other medical treatments. In Texas, we are licensed under The Texas Medical Board and adhere to strict cleanliness and safety standards. Acupuncture is a non-invasive, drug-free approach that works with your body's natural healing processes. It is not just for pain and ailments. Acupuncture can help keep you healthy and injury-free. Don't repeat my mistake of staying in pain for years when you can begin to feel better right now.

Acupuncture: A Pain Free Approach

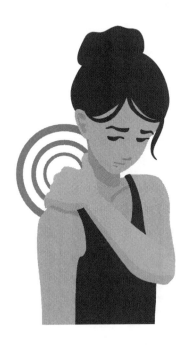

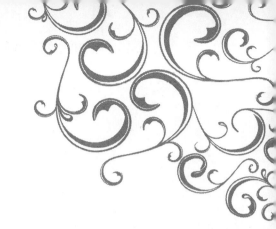

Part 1

What Is
Acupuncture?

Acupuncture: A Pain Free Approach

Let's start with the first two most common questions I get asked:
1. Does it hurt? No
2. Does it work? Yes

Acupuncture is part of a traditional Chinese medicinal practice that has been used for thousands of years to relieve hundreds of conditions. Its origins can be traced back to ancient Chinese provinces thousands of years ago. According to traditional Chinese medical texts, when Qi (pronounced 'Chee') flows freely throughout the body, we are healthy. When Qi is blocked, it can lead to pain, illness, and disease.

Healthy Qi is a way to describe being alive and well. It's not mystical. It is a beating heart. It is laughter. It is the force that gets you out of bed. A dysfunction in Qi leads to pain, fatigue and disease. Acupuncture is used to restore health and promote overall wellness. As you will see, this way of working with the body has been proven by many scientific studies.

Yin and Yang, Channels, Meridians, Kidney/Heart connection, tongue diagnosis, pulse diagnosis, excess and deficiency have a prominent and intrinsic link to Chinese medicine. Acupuncture school is an intense four years, too. In order to keep things easy to understand, I am addressing all of the intricacies of this medicine.

In my style of acupuncture, thin, sterile, single-use needles are placed into specific points on the body using a guide tube. The number of points varies depending on your specific condition. The acupuncture I practice is described in ancient texts that have not yet been translated into English. I had the honor of studying with the great Master Tan who brought this detailed and effective technique to the United States. I can offer pain relief in just one insertion.

I can put a needle in your ankle and relieve your neck pain. I can put one in your hand and relieve your back pain. This pain relief comes from treating the body as being a whole, single entity. At my first acupuncture session, I thought my acupuncturist was crazy putting needles in my ankle. There was a language barrier, and I felt the need to repeatedly remind him that I had shoulder pain and not ankle pain. He just patted my arm and motioned for me to lie back down.

I recently worked with a patient who had severe back pain. Unable to lie on his stomach because of a recent eye surgery, I had him lie on his back. He was confused and unsure of what I was going to do. Little did he know: two points in his wrist were all that was needed to reduce his pain in half. His pain was gone entirely after three more needles. It seemed like magic to him, as it does to many other patients who had never been exposed to this approach to medicine. My ability to do this comes from knowledge of people thousands of years ago. I have the honor of seeing miracles happen every day.

A Very Brief History of Acupuncture and Traditional Chinese Medicine
The earliest known text on acupuncture is the *Huang di Nei Jing,* or *Yellow Emperor's Inner Canon,* written sometime around 240 BC. This text describes the basic principles of acupuncture and provides a detailed description and location of acupuncture points. English translations are available, but it didn't make sense to me until someone who understood the Chinese language explained the nuances, beauty, and meaning behind every word and symbol.

Huang di Nei Jing contains two major texts, *Suwen* and *Lingshu.* They are structured as a series of conversations between the 'Yellow Emperor' (Huangdi) and his physician, commonly referred to as Qibo. The texts work together to bring us a complete explanation of Chinese medicinal theory, from diagnostic strategy to treatment methods.

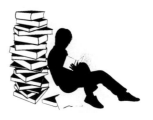

This book is a pivotal discovery and continues to inspire me to this day. It is profound learning directly from an ancient source and carry its teachings into the modern world. The techniques practitioners used successfully eons ago are available to me. Some historians even believe that methods of acupuncture date as far back to the Stone Age, where sharpened stones were used to drain abscesses or direct blood flow to an area to encourage healing. It is an ancient knowledge, and I consider it a privilege to have access to use it every day to help people.

Acupuncture: A Pain Free Approach

Acupuncture began to spread beyond China's borders in the sixth century AD, and was brought to Korea and Japan. But it was not until the twentieth century that acupuncture gained wider acceptance in the western world. In 1971, New York Times reporter James Reston wrote about his experience with acupuncture while on a trip to China. He had an emergency appendectomy and received acupuncture while in the hospital. After healing, he stayed to learn how these little needles were helping ill patients avoid medications. His article sparked an interest in acupuncture that continues to grow. It has been the fastest- growing medical treatment in the U.S. for decades.

Today, acupuncture is recognized as safe and effective, and is practiced all over the world. I worked on cruise ships for three years educating people on acupuncture and performing treatments. Sometimes I would do more than one hundred acupuncture sessions a week. Travelers kept coming back because they could enjoy their vacation without pain.

So...How Does it Work?

The foundation of acupuncture is difficult to grasp because it requires us to open our minds to a new way of seeing the body. Acupuncture highlights the interconnectedness of our body. The wrist can be used to relieve back pain. The foot can be used to relieve neck pain. Typically, your cardiologist doesn't help with back pain and your neurologist doesn't help with your knee pain. When you come into my office we talk about everything because your migraine may be connected to your digestion, your stress or something else. Two people with different issues may receive a similar treatment and two people with the same pain may receive completely different treatments. Acupuncture is customized. One size does not fit all.

Acupuncture stimulates specific points on the body which are believed to be channels through which Qi and blood flow. By inserting fine, sterile needles (about the width of a hair) into these points the body's natural healing process is stimulated.

Acupuncture needles are extremely thin and are made of stainless steel. Insertion into the skin is painless, with most patients reporting no discomfort during the treatment. Many people fall asleep while I am placing needles, and most fall asleep during the session. Once the needles are inserted, they are left in place for anywhere from ten to forty minutes.

During the treatment, a patient may experience a sensation of heaviness, warmth, or tingling around the needle site. This sensation, known as De Qi, is a sign that the needle has successfully stimulated the acupuncture point.

Thanks to the success of acupuncture around the world, many scientific studies have been conducted to help us understand how it works. These studies have shown that acupuncture releases the body's natural painkillers, such as enkephalin, and that it can help to reduce inflammation, improve circulation by increased oxygenation of tissue, and stimulate the immune system with increased white blood cell activity. Dopamine and serotonin were also observed in higher quantities.

- Data from twelve studies (8,003 participants) showed acupuncture was more effective than no treatment for back or neck pain. The pain-relieving effect of acupuncture was comparable to that of nonsteroidal anti-inflammatory drugs (NSAIDs).
- A clinical practice guideline from the American College of Physicians included acupuncture among the nondrug options recommended as first-line treatment for chronic low-back pain. Acupuncture is also one of the treatment options recommended for acute low-back pain.
- Data from 10 studies (2,413 participants) showed acupuncture was more effective than no treatment for osteoarthritis pain. Most of the participants in these studies had knee osteoarthritis, but some had hip osteoarthritis. The pain-relieving effect of acupuncture was comparable to that of NSAIDs.
- A clinical practice guideline from the American College of Rheumatology and the Arthritis Foundation conditionally recommends acupuncture for osteoarthritis of the knee, hip, or hand.
- More insurance companies are including acupuncture sessions to their plans since it is more cost effective than surgery.

Acupuncture works for pain.

Acupuncture: A Pain Free Approach

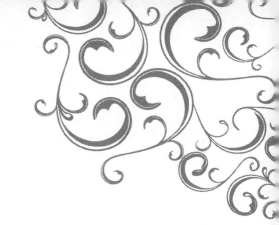

Part 2

The Benefits of Acupuncture

Acupuncture: A Pain Free Approach

The Benefits of Acupuncture

The abundance of scientific interest in acupuncture has confirmed the benefits of acupuncture are real. Some of the areas of research are in pain management, reducing stress and anxiety, improving sleep, reducing inflammation, reducing side effects of radiation from chemotherapy, and improving fertility.

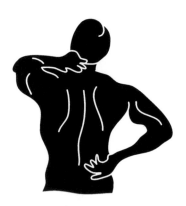

Pain Management

Acupuncture has been shown to be effective in treating both acute and chronic pain. Blood tests show an increase in the body's natural anti-inflammatory, pain relieving, and white blood cell activity. Some of the pain relievers that were observed to increase is called enkephalin. Enkephalin attaches to opioid receptors and has a pain-relieving effect stronger than morphine.

According to a 2017 study published in the *Journal of Pain Research,* acupuncture was found to be effective in reducing pain in patients with chronic low back pain. Other studies have found that acupuncture can help reduce pain in conditions such as osteoarthritis, migraines, and fibromyalgia.

Reducing Stress and Anxiety

A 2013 study published in the *Journal of Endocrinology* found that acupuncture helped to reduce stress hormone levels in patients with chronic stress. A 2018 study published in the *Journal of Alternative and Complementary Medicine* found that acupuncture was effective in reducing symptoms of anxiety in patients with generalized anxiety disorder.

Improving Sleep

Acupuncture has been found to be helpful in improving sleep quality. A 2018 study published in the journal *Evidence-Based Complementary and Alternative Medicine* found that acupuncture was effective in reducing insomnia symptoms in patients with chronic insomnia. Other studies have found that acupuncture can improve sleep quality in patients with other conditions, such as restless leg syndrome and sleep apnea.

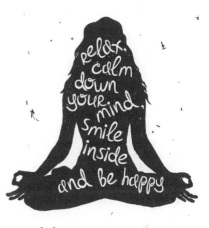

Reducing Inflammation

A 2018 study published in Brain, Behavior, and Immunity found that acupuncture helped to reduce inflammation in patients with rheumatoid arthritis. Other studies have found that acupuncture can help reduce inflammation in conditions such as asthma and irritable bowel syndrome.

Improving Fertility

Acupuncture has been found to be an effective treatment for improving fertility. A 2017 study published in the *Journal of Acupuncture and Meridian Studies* found that acupuncture improved pregnancy rates in patients undergoing in vitro fertilization. Other studies have found that acupuncture can improve sperm quality in men and regulate menstrual cycles in women.

Reducing Side Effects of Cancer Treatment

A 2018 study published in the *Journal of the National Cancer Institute* found that acupuncture helped to reduce joint pain in women undergoing aromatase inhibitor therapy for breast cancer. Other studies have found that acupuncture can help reduce nausea and vomiting in patients undergoing chemotherapy. I have patients who have found acupuncture helpful in chemotherapy-induced neuropathy.

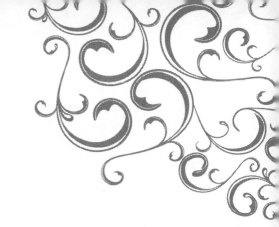

Part 3

What to Expect at Your Appointment

Acupuncture: A Pain Free Approach

My acupuncture sessions begin with a consultation to discuss your areas of concern and treatment options. You will fill out an online intake form similar to one you may fill out at any other doctor's office.

Upon arrival and for each session thereafter we will discuss your changes to your health and condition and the areas of focus for that day. Depending on where the needles will be placed, you may keep your clothes on or you may disrobe and cover yourself with a sheet. Heated table warmers and red-light heaters may be used therapeutically or to keep you warm and comfortable. I recommend you drink and eat something and use the restroom before arriving.

Thin, sterile, single-use needles will be placed into specific points on your body, using a guide tube. The number of needles used will vary depending on the focus for your specific needs. Once the needles are inserted, you will be relaxing for twenty to forty minutes. I have worked with many people that have a fear of needles. I always let them know that if they are uncomfortable for any reason throughout the session, I will remove the needle immediately, end the session at no cost; in almost twenty years of practice, I have never had a client take me up on this.

While you should never be tense or feel pain during your session, there are common sensations while the needles are inserted. You may experience sensations, like heaviness, warmth, and relaxation that surprise you. Please communicate any concerning sensation so you can be completely relaxed and comfortable. No pain, no gain does not apply in my clinic.

After the needles are inserted it is time to relax. It is not uncommon to feel a little groggy during the session because you are so relaxed; this feeling will cease as soon as you get up and move around. Sleepiness is due to the effect acupuncture sessions have in helping put your body in a 'rest and recovery' state. Your body may not be used to being in recovery mode because of stress or pain that occupies most of your daily life. Your body loves being in this recovery state and may take a minute to refocus.

Relaxing offers the best chance for you to receive the full benefit of your appointment. While I often leave the room, I will always check on you every ten minutes to make sure you are comfortable and see if you have any questions. Of course, I am also happy to stay in the room with a patient as long as necessary.

Once the session is over, the needles will be removed. The removal process is quick and your day can resume as normal following the session. I may perform cupping using my special technique (no bruising like Gwyneth Paltrow or swimmer Michael Phelps) and apply topical herbs to further improve healing and reduce pain. I recommend drinking plenty of water throughout the day of your appointment.

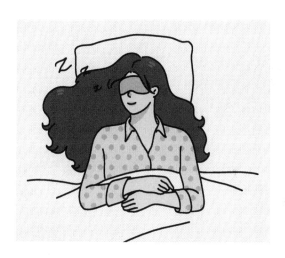

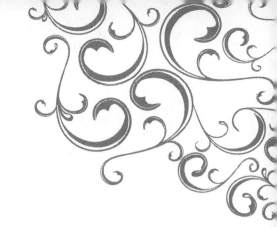

Part 4

Micro-Needling for Scars and Wrinkles

Acupuncture: A Pain Free Approach

I have recently fallen in love with the benefits of this style of acupuncture. It is a minimally invasive technique that has been proven to stimulate stem cell activity and collagen production. The results are incredible and my patients are very happy with their results. I've worked with people to reduce the appearance of surgical scars, acne scars, burn scars, and facial wrinkles. People with any skin tone can experience benefits, since it targets collagen and stem cell activity, not melanin.

Like acupuncture, micro-needling also has ancient roots. I use a medical-grade, state-of-the-art micro-needling device to painlessly stimulate collagen production and promote the skin's natural healing process. The device I use has been FDA-cleared and clinically proven to be safe and effective for all skin types.

This practice has gained popularity in recent years, mostly for its effectiveness in treating scars and wrinkles. Also known as collagen induction therapy, micro-needling involves creating tiny punctures in the skin's surface, which naturally stimulates the production of collagen and elastin, the two essential proteins for skin health and healing. When performed properly, the needles do not cause bleeding or any further scarring.

Improvements are usually noticeable within four or five sessions. Many people tell me friends and family make comments about improved appearance and glowing skin. Smoother texture and reduction in scar appearance are often seen after the first few sessions. Balanced skin tone, and a general brightness and youthful look to the skin is visible after every session.

Micro-needling is particularly effective for treating scars because it can penetrate the skin's top layer, which is where scars form. The procedure can improve the appearance of fine lines, wrinkles, various types of scars, including surgical scars, acne scars, stretch marks, and hyperpigmentation. A teenage patient of mine noticed improvements to the texture and redness of his acne scars within two session. His sister even reached out to tell me how happy his family is with the results.

Sessions are monthly and can be combined with your regular acupuncture session. Micro-needling session stake around fifty minutes. A topical numbing agent is used, which makes the treatment relatively pain-free, but it has been described as a slight stinging by some of my patients.

Your skin may remain pink for a couple of hours following your session. I always send my patients home with aftercare instructions and a custom blend to apply generously for the first couple of days. I also request that you don't wash your face with soap or wear makeup for the first eight hours. Keep your skin clean and open to absorb all the benefits of the topical blend.

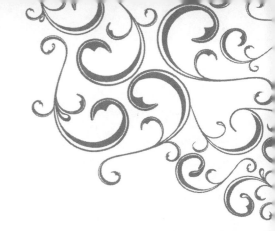

Frequently Asked Questions

Acupuncture: A Pain Free Approach

There are many misconceptions regarding acupuncture. I've been asked some wild questions: Do I dip the needles in medication? No. Do I chant, burn incense, or do a spiritual dance? No.

Acupuncture remains a mystery to many people and there is a lot of curiosity surrounding how it works, why it works, how much schooling it takes, and more. Here are some common questions that I receive:

Does it hurt?

Only one person in the thousands I have treated experienced significant pain. Even so, she continued to come in for five sessions because it relieved her thumb pain completely. I think most acupuncturists will end a session with no charge to you if you find the needles too uncomfortable to bear. I've had that policy in-place for years and no one has ever taken me up on it.

It can feel like a pinch, but most of the needles will be completely painless. I've had patients tell me they feel their muscles relax once the needle is in, and they sometimes say that the area feels cold or warm or swirling. I can adjust any needle if you feel it is uncomfortable.

Does it work?

Acupuncture Works!

Acupuncture has been around for a long time. Conservative estimates put acupuncture at around two thousand years old. Acupuncture continues to be one of the fastest-growing health modalities used by people to reduce a variety of symptoms. What doesn't work doesn't last!

Chinese Medicine hasn't grown because of mass marketing; the number of people receiving acupuncture grows because people share their experience. I continue to have a full practice because what I'm doing helps people feel better.

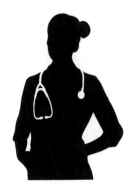

Today, most major hospitals have acupuncturists on staff, including: Johns

Hopkins, MD Anderson, Cleveland Clinic, Baylor Health, Children's Hospital, Memorial Sloan Kettering, and many more.

Where are needles inserted?
Needles can be inserted almost anywhere on your body. However, the most common areas are arms, legs, and back. When I was in school, we were required to have needled almost all of the three-hundred and fifty main acupuncture points.

Do needles go into nerves?
No!

Do you reuse the needles?
No, never. Once I remove them, I place them in a biohazard container.

Do needles go in the eyes?
I do not put a needle in eyes. I have heard of a technique that involves needle insertion close to the eye when working with glaucoma patients. I am not trained in this technique, but I did meet Andy Rosenfarb, MTOM, Dipl. Ac., Dipl. C.H., at an acupuncture seminar. He is an acupuncturist located in New Jersey who specializes in working with severe eye disorders, and he has reported the technique to be painless and effective.

Can acupuncture help me lose weight?
Patients have reported reduced cravings, improved digestion, reduced bloating, increased satiety, improved mood, and increased energy.

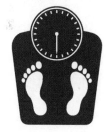

Is there medicine on the needles
No!

Can I get acupuncture if I'm pregnant?
Yes, and many women have found that acupuncture helps them have less pain, less nausea, less morning sickness, and a more comfortable pregnancy.

Acupuncture: A Pain Free Approach

Does acupuncture work for fertility, menopause and women's issues?
Many women have found success in improving their fertility, balancing their hormones, and regulating their periods using acupuncture and Chinese herbs.

Can acupuncture help me quit smoking?
People report that acupuncture was very helpful in reducing cravings and giving them a greater sense of calm, which helped them to quit smoking.

How many needles will you use?
This depends on how many areas are needing relief. For example, there are just a few points on the hand that relieve lower back pain.

How many appointments will I need?
It is impossible to look at someone and know exactly how many sessions they will need. The number of acupuncture sessions required will depend on several different factors, including the area being treated and the severity of the condition. Age is not necessarily a determining factor. In fact, I had a ninety-two-year-old woman come to see me for knee pain that had bothered her for more than thirty years and shoulder pain that had bothered her for ten years. The knee pain was relieved in one session. The shoulder pain took four months of treatments.

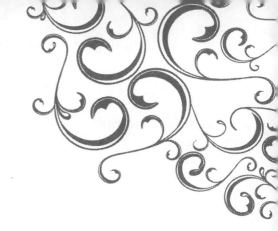

Related
Research

Back Pain

From: *National Library of Medicine*

In the first German trial patients with lower back pain (LBP) p(n=1,162) were randomized to either acupuncture treatments, placebo acupuncture treatments or optimal mainstream care. At 6 months, the primary endpoint, the proportion of positive clinical response was 47.6% with acupuncture, 44.2% with placebo acupuncture, and 27.4% with conventional care. There was no statistical difference between acupuncture and placebo acupuncture (p=0.39), but both acupuncture and placebo acupuncture were statistically and clinically superior to mainstream care that included physiotherapy, exercises and non-steroidal anti- inflammatory drugs (p<0.001).

Neck pain

From: *Journal of the American Medical Association*

Results: In the primary analysis, including all eligible randomized control trials (RCTs), acupuncture was superior to both sham and no-acupuncture control for each pain condition (P < .001 for all comparisons). After exclusion of an outlying set of RCTs that strongly favored acupuncture, the effect sizes were similar across pain conditions. Patients receiving acupuncture had less pain, with scores that were lower than those receiving sham acupuncture for back and neck pain, osteoarthritis, and chronic headache. Sham acupuncture is essentially fake acupuncture. These results were robust to a variety of sensitivity analyses, including those related to publication bias.

Conclusions: Acupuncture is effective for the treatment of chronic pain and is therefore a reasonable referral option. Significant differences between true and sham acupuncture indicate that acupuncture is more than a placebo.

Sciatica

From: *National Institute of Health National Library of Medicine*
This is a systematic review and meta-analysis, which aimed to assess the current evidence on the effects and safety of acupuncture for treating sciatica. In this review, a total of 11 randomized controlled trials were included. As a result, we found that the use of acupuncture may be more effective than drugs and may enhance the effect of drugs for patients with sciatica.

From: UTSW (UT Southwestern Medical Center)
https://www.utsouthwestern.edu/education/medical-school/departments/radiology/divisions-sections/community/population-health/briefs/acp-bk-rec.html

"ACP Recommends First Trying Nondrug Therapies for Back Pain"
September 19, 2017

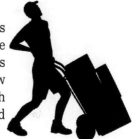

Earlier this year, the American College of Physicians (ACP) released an evidence-based clinical practice guideline (annals.org) that recommends physicians treat patients' non-radicular acute or subacute low back pain with non-pharmacologic therapies such as superficial heat, massage, acupuncture and spinal manipulation.

Researchers found that evidence did not support use of acetaminophen, which didn't improve pain outcomes versus a placebo. Low-quality evidence showed systemic steroids also weren't effective in treating acute or subacute low back pain.

For patients with chronic low back pain, the new ACP guidance recommends that physicians help patients initially select non-drug therapy with exercise, multidisciplinary rehabilitation, acupuncture, mindfulness- based stress reduction, tai chi, yoga, motor control exercise, progressive relaxation, electromyography biofeedback, low-level laser therapy, operant therapy, cognitive behavioral therapy, or spinal manipulation.

Acupuncture: A Pain Free Approach

Randomized Controlled Trial
Journal of Clinical Psychiatry, 2018 Dec 11;80(1):18m12235. doi: 10.4088/JCP.18m12235.

Acupuncture for Treatment of Persistent Disturbed Sleep: A Randomized Clinical Trial in Veterans With Mild Traumatic Brain Injury and Post traumatic Stress Disorder

Wei Huang 1 2 3, Theodore M Johnson 4 5, Nancy G Kutner 3, Sean N Halpin 6, Paul Weiss 7, Patricia C Griffiths 4, Donald L Bliwise 8

Conclusions: Real acupuncture, compared with a sham needling procedure, resulted in a significant improvement in sleep measures for veterans with mTBI and disturbed sleep, even in the presence of PTSD. These results indicate that an alternative-medicine treatment modality like acupuncture can provide clinically significant relief for a particularly recalcitrant problem affecting large segments of the veteran population.

From: Acupuncture in Medicine, April 2018
Acupuncture for lumbar disc herniation: a systematic review and meta-analysis
Shujie Tang 1, Zhuomao Mo 1, Renwen Zhang

Thirty RCTs involving 3503 participants were included in the study. Meta-analysis showed that acupuncture had a higher total effective rate than lumbar traction.

Conclusions: Acupuncture showed a more favorable effect in the treatment of LDH than lumbar traction, ibuprofen, diclofenac sodium, meloxicam, mannitol plus dexamethasone and mecobalamin, fugui gutong capsule plus ibuprofen, mannitol plus dexamethasone, loxoprofen

Acupuncture for Chronic Pain
Individual Patient Data Meta-analysis
Andrew J. Vickers, DPhil; Angel M. Cronin, MS; Alexandra C. Maschino, BS; et al

Our results from individual patient data meta-analyses of nearly 18 000 randomized patients in high-quality RCTs provide the most robust evidence to date that acupuncture is a reasonable referral option for patients with chronic pain.

Johns Hopkins Medicine
Quoted directly from their website: https://www.hopkinsmedicine.org/health/wellness-and-prevention/acupuncture

How does acupuncture affect the body?
Acupuncture points are believed to stimulate the central nervous system. This, in turn, releases chemicals into the muscles, spinal cord, and brain. These biochemical changes may stimulate the body's natural healing abilities and promote physical and emotional well-being.

National Institutes of Health (NIH) studies have shown that acupuncture is an effective treatment alone or in combination with conventional therapies to treat the following:
- Nausea caused by surgical anesthesia and cancer chemotherapy
- Dental pain after surgery
- Addiction
- Headaches
- Menstrual cramps
- Tennis elbow
- Fibromyalgia
- Myofascial pain
- Osteoarthritis
- Low back pain
- Carpal tunnel syndrome
- Asthma

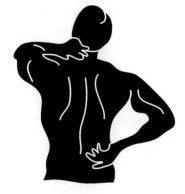

It may also help with stroke rehabilitation.
A note from Cleveland Clinic (https://my.clevelandclinic.org/health/treatments/4767-acupuncture)

Acupuncture: A Pain Free Approach

We're only beginning to understand the effects of acupuncture. Research stories from people who've tried it have shown that it may help alleviate some illnesses and symptoms. If you decide to try acupuncture, check your practitioner's credentials first to be sure they're qualified, experienced and use good sanitation practices.

MD Anderson website (https://www.mdanderson.org/patients-family/diagnosis-treatment/care-centers-clinics/integrative-medicine-center/clinical-services.html)
Acupuncture is a nearly 2,000-year-old form of traditional Chinese medicine. In acupuncture, thin needles are inserted through the skin at specific points on the body. In combination with conventional treatments, studies indicate acupuncture may be beneficial for several conditions, including chemotherapy-induced nausea and vomiting, cancer and treatment-related pain, peripheral neuropathies, dry mouth, hot flashes, fatigue and stress management.

Excerpts from National Institutes of Health

"Research Progress on the Mechanism of the Acupuncture Regulating Neuro-Endocrine-Immune Network System"
Jingwen Cui,[1,2,†] Wanrong Song,[1,2,†] Yipeng Jin,[1,†] Huihao Xu,[1] Kai Fan,[1] Degui Lin,[1] Zhihui Hao,[1,2,*] and Jiahao Lin[1,2,*]
Tomohiro Yonezawa, Academic Editor

The current research about acupuncture's effects on local skin immunity mainly focuses on the interaction between immune cells, immune molecules, free nerve endings, the activation of the nervous system and local HPA axis, etc. In terms of the research on the effects of acupuncture on psoriasis, Wang et al. [131] demonstrated that electroacupuncture improved skin lesions, decreased epidermal thickness, inhibited the proliferation of keratinocytes, and reduced CD3 T cell infiltration significantly. In addition, electroacupuncture decreased the secretion of inflammatory cytokines, including IL-1β, IL-17A and IL-23p40, and down-regulated the expression level of neurokinin A (NKA), which is correlated positively to the extent of decreased inflammatory cytokines in local lesions [131]

Previous studies of acupuncture on cellular immunity regulation established that it can regulate the number of T lymphocytes and their subsets, adjust the conversion rate of T lymphocytes, and also modulate the ratio of CD4/CD8 [109]. One of the primary mechanisms is the balanced tuning of Th1/Th2. In allergic rhinitis, bronchial asthma and chronic fatigue syndrome, acupuncture can reverse the Th1/Th2 balance in the direction of Th1 [110,111,112]. Conversely, while in depression and embryo implantation disorders, acupuncture can move the Th1/Th2 balance toward Th2 [113,114].

Acupuncture can exert brain-protective effects by regulating microglia. Microglia are glial cells, which are another kind of immune cell mainly located in the central nervous system. They are the first and most vital defense in the central nervous system. In the healthy brain, microglia work hard as "logistical cells" to clear dead cells and generate neurotrophic factors that immerse neurons in protective factors. A large number of clinical studies have proven that activated microglia play a dominant role in the pathogenesis of neurodegenerative diseases, such as Parkinson's disease, Alzheimer's disease and multiple sclerosis.

Acupuncture can stimulate the HPA axis to release endorphins that bind to the opioid receptors on the surface of NK cells and stimulate NK cells to increase the expression of cell adhesion molecules, granzyme B and perforin. Meanwhile, acupuncture intervenes in the regulation procedure of immunosuppression through NK cells. Studies have confirmed that the immune regulatory network, which is mainly composed of IL-2, IFN and NK cells, plays a crucial role in enhancing and regulating the body's immune function, which is inseparably intertwined with some pathological conditions such as tumorigenesis

Acupuncture can significantly enhance phagocytosis in pathological conditions or hypo-immunity. When the phagocytosis is hyperactive, acupuncture will down-regulate it to reduce the phagocytosis index. Current studies suggested that the regulatory effect may be associated with the activation of the cholinergic anti-inflammatory pathway (CAP) as well as the regulation of scavenger receptors' (SRs) expression and M1/M2 macrophage polarization.

Acupuncture can affect the immune system by regulating the neuroendocrine system. Meanwhile, acupuncture is also able to influence the neuroendocrine system by modulating the immune system.

Several studies have demonstrated that the therapeutic effects of acupuncture are related to the regulation of brain-gut peptides. Initially, SP has different physiological effects on the body. β-EP acts as one of the markers of changes in the body. It often predicted reduction in headache frequency when β-EP level is above 4 ng/mL in cerebrospinal fluid

Acetylcholine is the main neurotransmitter of the vagus nerve, which regulates the production of cytokines on a variety of immune cells by activating α7 nicotinic acetylcholine receptors (nAChRs) and promoting T cell development and/or differentiation [51]. Both nAChRs and muscarinic acetylcholine receptors (mAChRs) can regulate the synthesis and release of cytokines such as TNF-α, IFN-β and IL-6, thereby regulating immunity [6].

Studies have shown that acupuncture can increase the low level of acetylcholine in patients with Parkinson's disease and dementia as well as promote the production of acetylcholine in intracerebral hemorrhage rats with reduced acetylcholine release [52]. According to the research, acupuncture at GV-20 and K-11 in the treatment of Alzheimer's disease resulted in increased levels of plasma acetylcholine, which is one of the biological mechanisms [53]. In addition, the mechanism of acupuncture at BL-13 in the treatment of allergic asthma in rats is also related to the inhibition of the synthesis and release of acetylcholine

Studies have shown that acupuncture has a regulating effect on monoamine neurotransmitters. Acupuncture at DU-16 can improve the memory impairment of dementia mice by significantly increasing the contents of 5-HT, norepinephrine (NA) and dopamine (DA) in the brain tissue [48]. For intracerebral hemorrhagic rats with increased release of CA, acupuncture at PC-6, GV-26 and ST-9 can inhibit the release of CA [49]. Studies have proven that electroacupuncture can reduce the levels of the plasma monoamine neurotransmitters 5-HT, DA and NE to relieve anorexia in rats.

As benign stress, acupuncture can change the concentration of certain neurotransmitters, including monoamines and acetylcholine.

Acupuncture can regulate the release of neurotransmitters, neuropeptides, and hormones by stimulating the neuroendocrine system. In addition, acupuncture can also indirectly affect the immune system by regulating the neuroendocrine system, specifically embodying the substances released by the neuroendocrine system acting on the corresponding receptors of immune organs and immune cells.

Additionally, some recent studies have indicated that acupoints are distributed in areas of neuroimmune modulation. Histologically, acupoints are also found in high-density regions of mast cells, lymph-vessels and arteriovenous plexuses in addition to areas with concentrated innervation [37]. Immunohistochemistry and fluorescence microscopy has proven synaptic connections between mast cells and nerve endings [38]. Furthermore, the western blot test confirmed that transient receptor potential vanilloid subtype 2 (TRPV2) channel protein expression on the mast cell membrane. This channel could be activated by mechanical force and high temperature [39]. Thus, acupuncture or moxibustion can stimulate mast cells' degranulation and release of histamine, substances P and 5-HT, etc.

Acupuncture: A Pain Free Approach

From: *Neuroscience Letters,* May 6, 2004
"**Acupuncture and Endorphins**"

Ji-Sheng Han

Acupuncture and electroacupuncture (EA) as complementary and alternative medicine have been accepted worldwide mainly for the treatment of acute and chronic pain. Studies on the mechanisms of action have revealed that endogenous opioid peptides in the central nervous system play an essential role in mediating the analgesic effect of EA. Further studies have shown that different kinds of neuropeptides are released by EA with different frequencies. For example, EA of 2 Hz accelerates the release of enkephalin, beta-endorphin and endomorphin, while that of 100 Hz selectively increases the release of dynorphin. A combination of the two frequencies produces a simultaneous release of all four opioid peptides, resulting in a maximal therapeutic effect. This finding has been verified in clinical studies in patients with various kinds of chronic pain including low back pain and diabetic neuropathic pain.

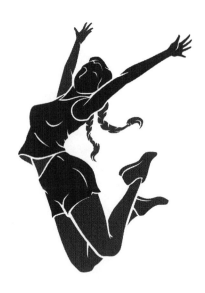

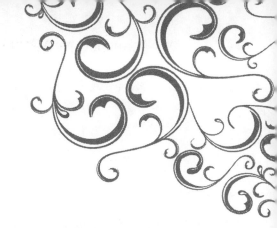

Testimonials

Acupuncture: A Pain Free Approach

I regularly receive testimonials from patients sharing with me know how successful their treatment has been. I'd like to share some of those with you.

Relief from Fear and Pain

From Olivia C.

If you've ever questioned the science of acupuncture or were afraid of needles; this review is for you. I am normally extremely averse to needles. Extremely. However, I have been told by multiple sources about Gail and the incredible work she performed. So, I found myself in a quandary; I had just recently done some damage to my knee, but I was days away from my tennis team playoffs. I didn't have a choice. I had to seek help and I had to suck up my fear of needles.

So, I called Gail.

Perhaps she knew how frightened I was; maybe she didn't. She talked me through each move she was about to do; none of that surprising popping stuff you get at the chiropractor. I've never understood how a needle in one place of your body could alleviate pain elsewhere but who am I to judge? After fifteen minutes of mild discomfort (seriously wish my doctors knew how to draw blood as painless as she worked her needles), multiple parts of my body had started releasing their tension. I can't explain it, just know I am a cynic who now believes. Tomorrow, I suit up for my team's playoff chances; a BIG thank you to Gail for that. I will be back.

From Cathy B.

Several car accidents have left me with severe chronic pain. I have tried everything to find relief from the constant pain. Some of the only relief I've found has been from Gail. If you know anyone who needs help with pain or stress management, I highly recommend they give Gail a call. For the first time in years, I have found someone who understands how to treat, and relieve my pain. Anyone living with chronic pain knows what an incredible feeling that is! When I'm dealing with someone that is treating my pain, I personally need them to be someone I can feel completely comfortable around. Gail is that person. The only thing that outshines her AMAZING personality is her professionalism, and magical needles! I would recommend her to anyone.

From M.P.

I would like to add my story to the testimonials. After several years of arthritis neck pain, I was in an auto accident which aggravated my symptoms. Additionally, I suffer from chronic sinus headaches. I decided to try acupuncture when I heard about Gail and I have been amazed at the level of relief that was achieved with just four treatments. Gail genuinely cares about her clients and offers not only professional treatments, but also support and encouragement. I highly recommend her services.

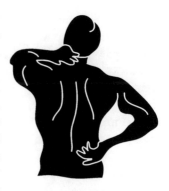

From Kelsey G.

Gail's knowledge and expertise are outmatched only by her empathy and care. She is an absolute gem and my quality of life has been infinitely improved by working with her. I have been seeing her for a year and a half now to help manage the inflammation in my body resulting from a few autoimmune diseases. As a result of Gail's treatments and some other life changes, I've been able to significantly reduce the amount of medications I've been taking. Her skills are invaluable and I feel so fortunate to have found her.

From Brooke M.

I had my first appointment with Gail this week. Having never done acupuncture before I was not sure what to expect. Gail was very welcoming and made me feel comfortable and relaxed. She is extremely compassionate and caring. She truly cares about your issues and concerns. I was able to easily voice all my thoughts and worries with her.

Acupuncture: A Pain Free Approach

For me, this appointment helped in more ways than just the acupuncture, it was therapeutic just to speak with her. I am looking forward to my next appointment and highly recommend Gail!

From Angie B.

I cannot rave enough about Gail. She is extremely knowledgeable and I felt so much better after treatments. I have seen her a few times and it is amazing how quickly your body resets itself. This is such a different and, in a way, simpler approach to achieving better health. I recommend a free consultation if you are hesitant. She is the real deal!

From Emily G.

I went in to see Gail for jaw pain that had been bothering me for about a week. I wasn't sure what the cause was but thought acupuncture could help. It only took one session with Gail to rid me of the pain. Now, six months later, I am still pain-free just like her business name implies. Five stars all the way!

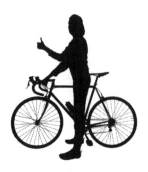

From Leslie S.

Gail has done so much for me. We made amazing progress with NATE allergy treatment. We improved my digestion, I lost inflammation and fifteen pounds. I knew right where to go when I had a biking injury. Massage, chiropractic and a trip to the orthopedic doctor didn't give me pain relief, but a few sessions with Gail gave me significant relief. I highly recommend her! -

From Cara B.

Gail is an amazing holistic practitioner. I have a herniated disc in my neck with numbness and tingling in my hand. She has been helping nerve issues with acupuncture. She recently acquired a HBOT hyperbaric oxygen therapy device.

I am trying this pure oxygen saturation treatment to help diminish nerve symptoms by increasing red blood cells to promote healing. I have only excellent things to say about Gail Daugherty. I referred several patients to her and they were all very pleased with the results.

From Donna S., Senior Clinical Physical Therapist

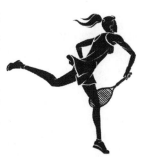

I felt that any patient referred to Gail would benefit from her expertise and often showed functional improvements which would enhance my therapy as well. She showed a tremendous knowledge of acupuncture and pain management. With the overwhelmingly positive feedback from my patients, I had several treatments myself and was very impressed with the outcome.

From P.J.

Gail has been a pleasant surprise introducing acupuncture to my healing process for my right knee. I have been impressed with her knowledge, approach and the calm that results after each treatment. She has not only helped comfort my knee, but each visit, I feel better overall. As an active competitor in multiple sports, I am convinced acupuncture will help my performance, help me maintain a high level of fitness, address injuries and even prevent them over time. I am looking forward to my continued weekly sessions as part of my wellness program. I highly recommend and many thanks to Gail at Pain Free Acupuncture Clinic.

From E.J.

Gail is an excellent acupuncturist and a great person. I have been using her services for a long time and have excellent results. She also helped out my daughter's stress last year before her wedding.

From A.P.

Thanks so much for relieving all of my aches and pains!

Acupuncture: A Pain Free Approach

From M.S.

Gail has wonderful energy! Very kind and knowledgeable. The treatment definitely got my circulation and energy flowing (read: a LOT)! Looking forward to more treatments!

From R.F.

After four weeks of treatments with Gail for my tendonitis is completely gone and I never skipped a day of tennis. It was amazing!

From V.K.

I sprained my left ankle really badly. I did all the normal things, like applying hot and cold, saw a chiropractor, did electrical treatments, but still I had a lot of pain and swelling and little mobility. Today my foot has no pain. My mobility is back.

From D.G

I highly recommend Gail. After only three sessions I am truly pain-free. Gail is very professional and caring.

From S.W

I no longer have migraines! I have had migraine headaches since 1978. It worked! I have not had a migraine or severe headache. You are professional, calm and caring in your demeanor. She listens carefully to what's going on in my life, thoughtfully processes, and then moves forward. I cannot thank her enough! I highly recommend her acupuncture services.

I also suffer from chronic pain and have for decades. I have had four back surgeries and one neck surgery. I have had three treatments. My pain is greatly diminished, as is my swelling and tightness. I cannot end this testimonial without a high amount of praise for Gail Daugherty. Her expertise, bedside manner, aura and spirit are instrumental in the experience and outcome of the treatment [a]

From C.W.

I had limited range of motion in left arm due to breakage of years previous. Compensation for pain perhaps caused right side and lower back and hip issues. In just that first session I could move my arm to the back of my head pain free!! She then moved to the right side where range of motion was already good but pain in lower back. Within minutes, pain free for first time in months. Do not think twice about trying this.

From E.G.

I went in to see Gail for jaw pain that had been bothering me for about a week. I wasn't sure what the cause was but thought acupuncture could help. It only took one session with Gail to rid me of the pain. Now, six months later, I am still pain-free just like her business name implies. Five stars all the way!

From G.L.

When I first saw Gail my right elbow was swollen and painful. By the final treatment the swelling had almost completely gone and I was having minimal discomfort – a vast improvement.

From T.J.

Gail is amazing! I have gotten acupuncture from many practitioners and Gail's treatments have by far been the most effective and enjoyable. She listens, explains exactly what is going to happen during the treatment, and has such a calm and soothing energy. She has helped me sleep better, eliminated my shoulder pain, and calmed me down during stressful times with her gentle techniques. I highly recommend her!

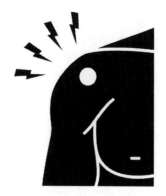

Acupuncture: A Pain Free Approach

From D.B.

I highly recommend Pain Free Acupuncture to anyone in the Dallas, Plano Mckinney, and surrounding area. Gail Daugherty is terrific, skilled, and an impressive healer.

My son sustained a knee injury while running cross-country in high school. The pain was so intense he was told he wouldn't recover. After working with Gail, his pain subsided and she was instrumental in motivating him to try again.

From C.W.

Gail is Awesome! She is so friendly, comfortable to talk to and really knows what she's talking about! I was a little weary at first about needles, but she explains everything and makes you feel very comfortable. I have chronic back pain and we were able to get my pain from a level eight to a level three just in the first treatment! This treatment really helps, so give it a try! Also, such a friendly front desk staff!

From Jessica G.

Gail is amazing! I have suffered from migraines for more than ten years and have tried everything from different medications to receiving Botox injections. Once seeing Gail and having acupuncture combined with her knowledge of Chinese herbs I can honestly say there has been such an improvement! I now only have one or two migraines a month compared to fifteen to twenty. If you suffer from migraines Gail is the person you need to see!

From C.T.

I have suffered from lower back pain for the last eight years. Even after one treatment with Gail my pain was significantly decreased and after my second treatment, it was gone. I would recommend acupuncture to anyone who doesn't want to suffer any longer.

From Gaye

I want to thank Gail so much for all her help and kindness. I have been walking without a limp and no hip pain.

From McG

Gail worked miracles for me! After my treatment my back pain decreased significantly. I returned to Gail when I experienced stomach upset. She again treated me and within hours I felt much better.

From D.P.

Even after the first treatment, I felt a vast improvement. The range of motion in my shoulder is back to normal. As a paraplegic I am completely dependent on the use of my shoulders, so I was very pleased with the treatment.

From M.E.

For anyone living with pain–get to Gail!! I had a severe sciatic episode and had to practically crawl into my appointment (which by the way was SO easy to schedule online!!). Afterward, I was almost entirely pain free, and by the next day, no pain at all. Truly amazing. Gail is highly professional and so empathetic, she is just awesome. I cannot recommend her highly enough! If I could give more than five stars, I absolutely would!

From Julia and Trevor

My husband and I have benefited from Gail's skills. I can now find a comfortable position in which to sleep, resulting in more restful nights. My back is much more flexible in the morning. We are both most grateful to Gail.

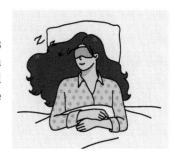

Acupuncture: A Pain Free Approach

From G. T.

Gail is friendly, knowledgeable, and provides excellent/top notch service as an acupuncture therapist. I tried acupuncture for minor back pain after several other types of treatment failed to improve/reduce the pain.

I was amazed at how quickly acupuncture worked, and within three treatments my pain was almost non-existent. Gail's approach to acupuncture is very patient focused; she is very thoughtful, answers questions in a friendly manner, and genuinely cares about the well-being of each person receiving treatment.

I would highly recommend her to anyone looking to try acupuncture therapy for pain, allergies, or general stress relief. Gail is the best!

From A.P.

Severe back, neck and shoulder problems go back several years. Have relied on osteopathy and physiotherapy before, but this was the first time ever tried acupuncture. Thanks to Gail am heading home virtually pain free.

From S.W.

I suffer from chronic pain and have for decades. I have had four back surgeries and one neck surgery. I have had three treatments. My pain is greatly diminished, as is my swelling and tightness. I cannot end this testimonial without a high amount of praise for Gail Daugherty. Her expertise, bedside manner, aura and spirit are instrumental in the experience and outcome of the treatment.

From J.C.

Gail's acupuncture has helped my painful knees. I am walking with improved mobility and less pain when walking up and down stairs.

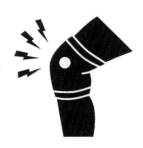

From G.L.

When I first saw Gail my right elbow was swollen and painful. By the final treatment the swelling had almost completely gone and I was having minimal discomfort – a vast improvement.

From A.B.

Gail Daugherty is an excellent acupuncturist and health practitioner. She is very knowledgeable about nutrition and explains everything clearly. I have seen her for several issues and I always feel listened to, comfortable and ultimately feel better after treatments. She also recommends Chinese herbs which are reasonably priced and effective. I definitely recommend her. I know she offers free consultations if you are hesitant or have questions.

As the knee is certainly on the mend, I have been so impressed with her knowledge and the calm she brings to every area of my body, mind and soul. She is a true healer.

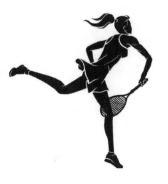

In just one session, Gail was able to relieve my upper neck and back stiffness! She also eradicated pain in my shins that I thought I would just have to live with. (I learned that the two are related in Chinese medicine/ acupuncture.) Gail must be able to channel her calm energy through her needles – often times at the end of my sessions, I don't want to get down from the cloud I'm on. In addition to her expertise in acupuncture, she studied with the founder of NAET (Nambudripad's Allergy Elimination Technique) and is helping to rid me of some annoying allergies that have plagued me for years. I highly recommend Dr. Daugherty who can also answer dietary questions since she also has her PhD in nutrition!

From Ivy

Gail - I am truly so grateful that I have been able to meet you. What a miracle it was that you practice close enough to where I have severed my ENTIRE mission so far!! I am truly so grateful for the privilege of knowing you!!

Acupuncture: A Pain Free Approach

You are the coolest person ever and you have become one of my dearest friends. I love that you are always seeking to know more in life. I love how much you seek after truth, and wisdom, and everything that is good. I can feel how deep your gratitude to Him is, in everything you say and do. You have become a beacon of light, cheerfulness, and hope to me, and I have truly felt edified and uplifted each and every time we have been able to talk. I am forever grateful for the physical and spiritual healing that has taken place in your office for me.

From A.G.

I went to Gail for acupuncture for sciatica constant pain, nasal congestion and for digestive problems. My breathing has gotten 85 percent better. My intestine has resumed being regular. My sciatica has been killing me for four to five years and is now 50 percent better. I shall resume treatment when I get back home in order to get rid of it completely.

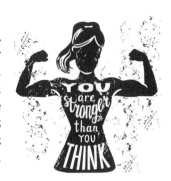

From S.W.

I no longer have migraines! I have had migraine headaches since 1978. It worked! I have not had a migraine or severe headache. Gail is professional, calm and caring in her demeanor. She listens carefully to what's going on in my life, thoughtfully processes and then moves forward. I cannot thank her enough! I highly recommend her acupuncture services.

From A.D

I had lower back pain and sciatic pain in my leg. I had just had back epidurals six weeks prior but still felt pain. Gail's treatments took 99 percent of all discomfort away. In addition, I have pronounced allergies and allergic rhinitis. Gail worked on these so that I could breathe better and the GI symptoms improved dramatically. For the first time my food allergies seemed reduced – my stomach was no longer bloated. My husband even noticed that my spirits were lifted. I had more energy and a brighter spirit as I was free of pain.

From L.S.

Gail has done so much for me. We made amazing progress with NATE allergy treatment. Improved my digestion, I lost inflammation and fifteen pounds. I knew right where to go when I had a biking injury. Massage, chiropractic and a trip to the orthopedist didn't give me pain relief but a few sessions with Gail gave me significant relief. I highly recommend her!

From L.K.

After I had my son via Cesarean I began to suffer from bloating and severe constipation. I had colonics which provided temporary relief, but soon after my condition would return. I began to watch my fiber intake, started taking a fiber supplement, exercised more, drank lots of water, used laxatives, took probiotics and nothing worked.

Finally out of desperation I decided to try acupuncture after watching a segment about it on The Today Show. I consulted with Gail Daugherty at The Cooper Center in McKinney (sic) and we worked out a flexible plan for me to receive four thirty minute sessions every Friday more a month. After the first treatment I felt some relief. Then after the second I felt more relief. After the third, more.

Four sessions into it I feel so much better and definitely feel that acupuncture played an important part in my recovery.

From Oscar S.

I am a college baseball pitcher and we go through long and grueling seasons. I have been going to Gail for three years now and she has single handedly saved my season when cortisone shots and other pain treatments couldn't help me. She has become my go to pain management before and after every season and has helped keep me healthy so I could achieve things such as winning a conference title and setting a personal milestone of throwing 72 innings in a single season. I highly recommend coming here if you are an athlete looking to get healthy or someone who is struggling with nagging pain or injuries.

Acupuncture: A Pain Free Approach

From C.T.

Gail has been amazing! We are convinced acupuncture was a big part of healing our daughter's stress fracture. Her sports related injury has a low healing percentage.

From K.M., age 17

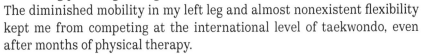

For the past three years, I have been dealing with chronic hamstring pain originating from a series of muscle tears. The diminished mobility in my left leg and almost nonexistent flexibility kept me from competing at the international level of taekwondo, even after months of physical therapy.

After just one session of acupuncture, the results were drastic. I could stretch my left leg almost without pain. In the ensuing sessions, my results never ceased to amaze me, as more and more improvement followed each treatment. The flexibility in my left leg surpasses that of my right leg! Hopefully now I'll be able to compete in Olympic team trials; because of acupuncture, I now have no physical limitations.

From P.J.

Pain Free Acupuncture Clinic is now a great part of my weekly routine. Gail has introduced me to what I consider to be a key part of my health and wellness. She began with her specialized healing process with needles to help pain associated with a dislocated patella in my right knee. As the knee is certainly on the mend, I have been so impressed with her knowledge and the calm she brings to every area of my body, mind and soul. She is a true healer.

As an active competitor in multiple sports, I am convinced acupuncture needs to be a part of my performance prep. Gail and her approach is helping me maintain a high level of fitness, address injuries and prevent them over time. I look forward to continuing my weekly sessions as part of my overall wellness program. I highly recommend Pain Free Acupuncture Clinic and many thanks to Gail for helping me feel great!

Please let me know of any editing errors, how to add your name to the growing list of testimonials, and to experience pain and stress relief.

Contact:
www.PainFreeGailID.com
BeInspired@PainFreeGailID.com

I look forward to working with you to give you the care you need to live your best life.

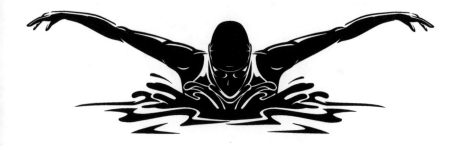

Meet the Author

Gail Daugherty is not your average acupuncturist. With a diverse background and a thriving practice, she has established herself as the go-to expert for pain relief in the Dallas area. But her journey to success is anything but ordinary.

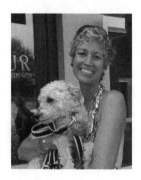

She perfected her techniques while living and learning from experts around the world. Learning and enjoying the adventure of working in reality television, teaching Biochemical Nutrition, and becoming a visiting acupuncturist on cruise lines. She honed her skills, followed her heart, and built her practice near her parents in North Dallas. In no time, she became known as one of the best in the field, catching the attention of none other than Dr. Kenneth Cooper, a renowned figure in preventative medicine.

Gail's achievements don't stop there. She is a Board Certified Acupuncturist, holds a PhD in Holistic Nutrition, is a published author, and has earned an MBA and a Master of Acupuncture and Chinese Medicine.

Gail's genuine care and passion to help is what sets her apart. She works closely with you to relieve your pain and stress. Her unique methods build on ancient medicine and modern techniques, offering you the opportunity to feel your best.

Please contact her with any questions at BeInspired@PainFreeGailD.com

Made in the USA
Columbia, SC
19 November 2024

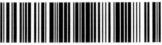

46422079R00035